THIS BOOK BELONGS TO

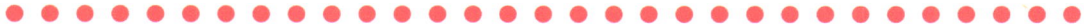

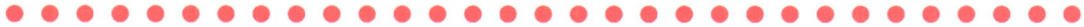

••

••

This book is for all the wonder mommies and chronic illness warriors everywhere. Stay Strong!

Library of Congress Control Number: 2020922485
ISBN: 978-1-7328263-5-9

WONDER MOMMY

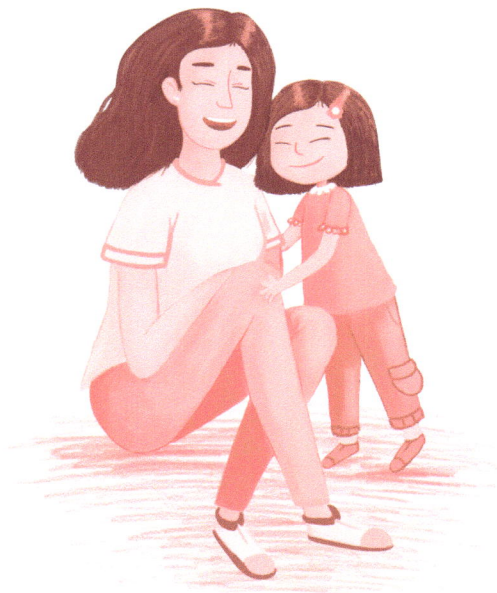

Jennifer Senne

Andreea Balcan

Mommy loves to spend time with me.
We dance and sing!

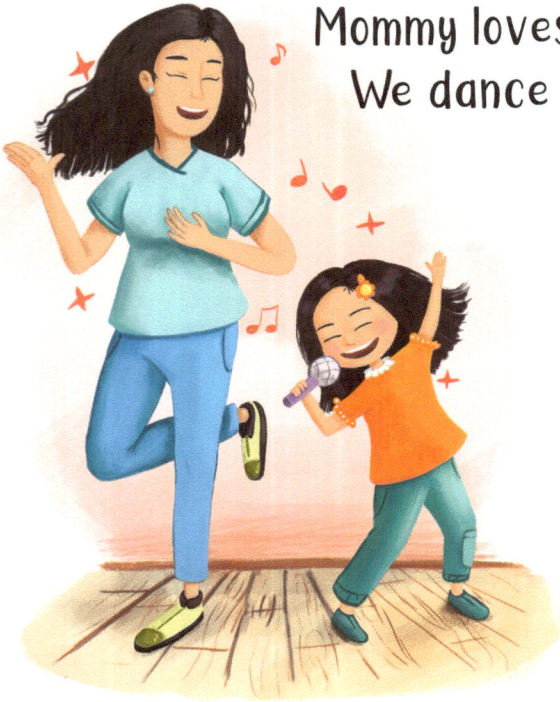

We ride our bikes!

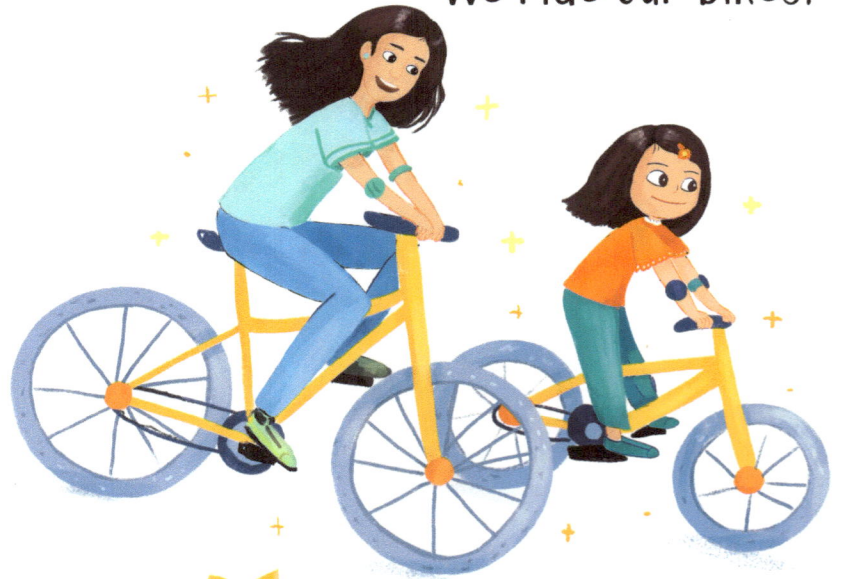

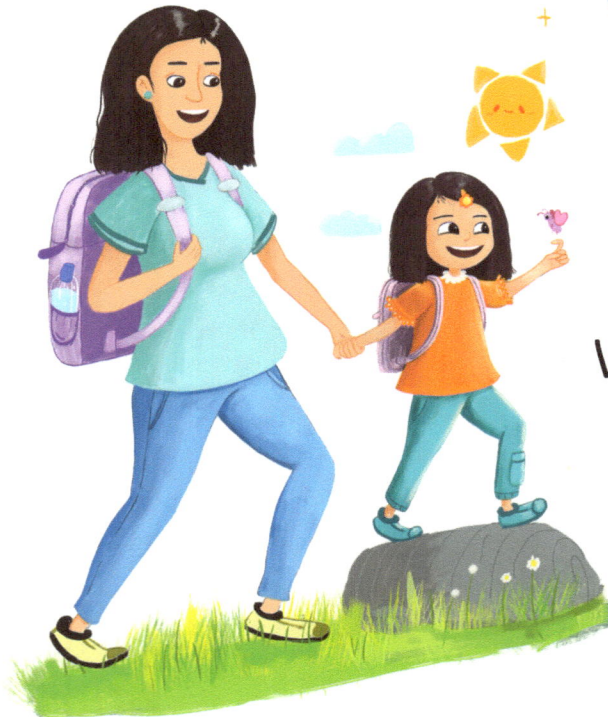

We swim and swing!
We go for hikes!

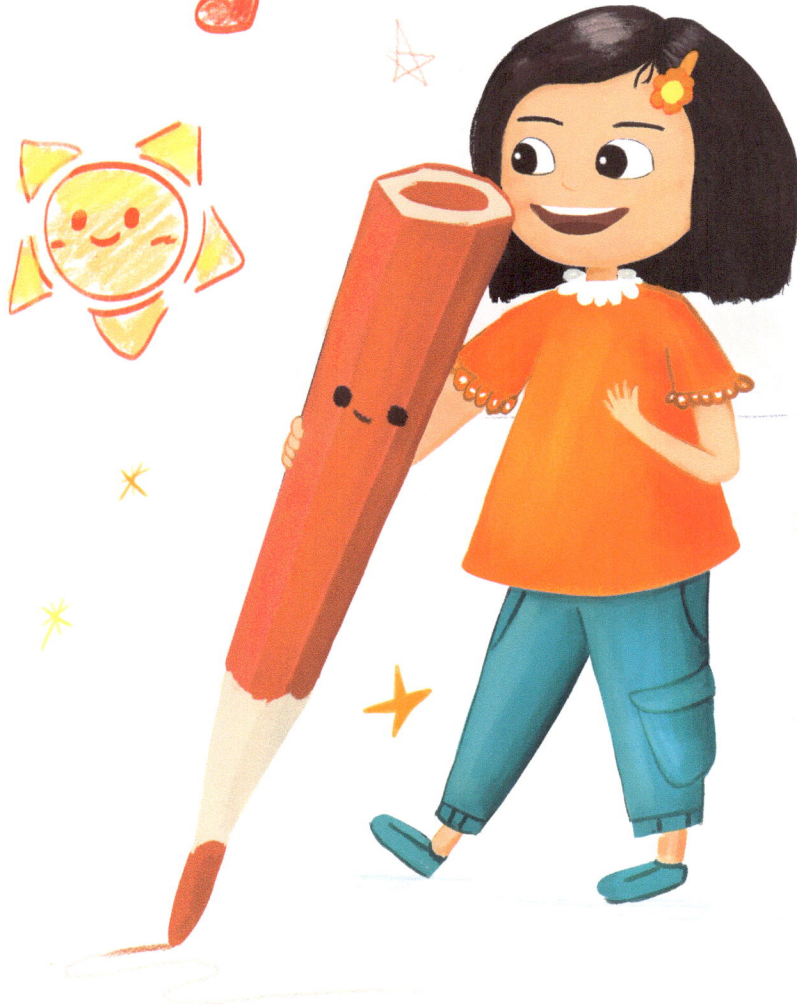

She's my Wonder Mommy!

Sometimes it's hard for Mommy to move around.
Sometimes she can't walk, but we can still have fun!

We watch a show!
We make some art!
We play with dough!
We draw a heart!

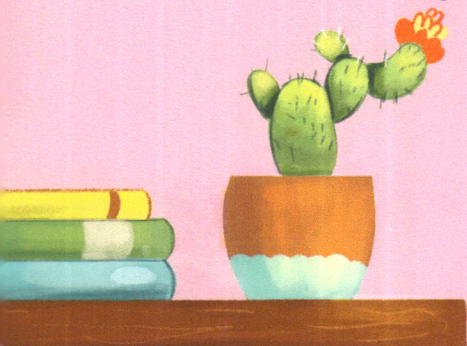

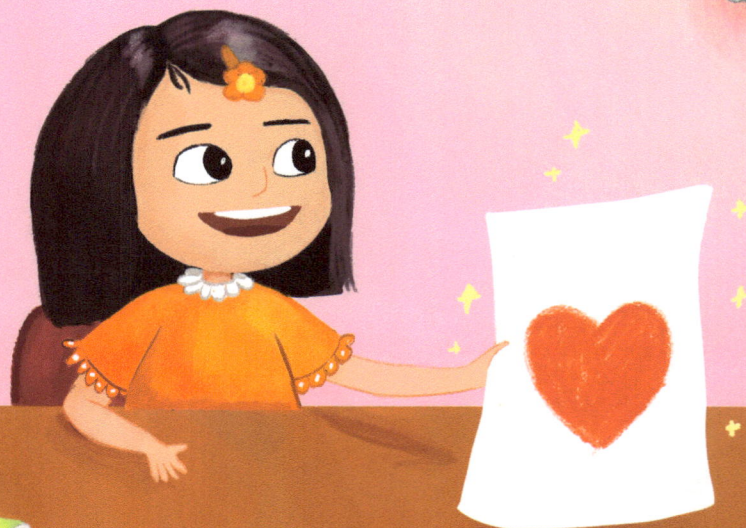

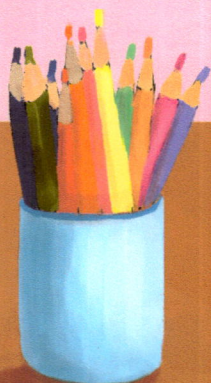

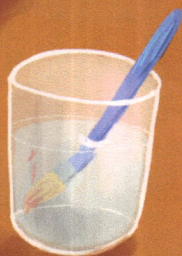

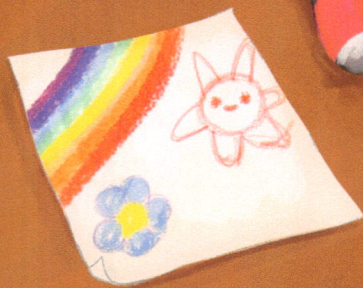

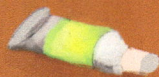

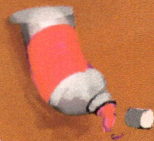

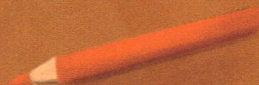

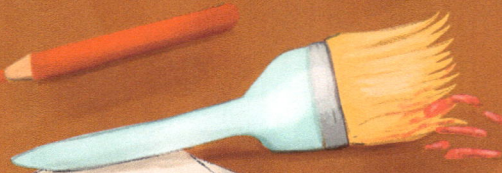

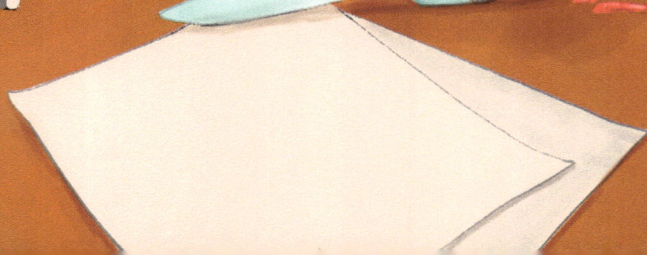

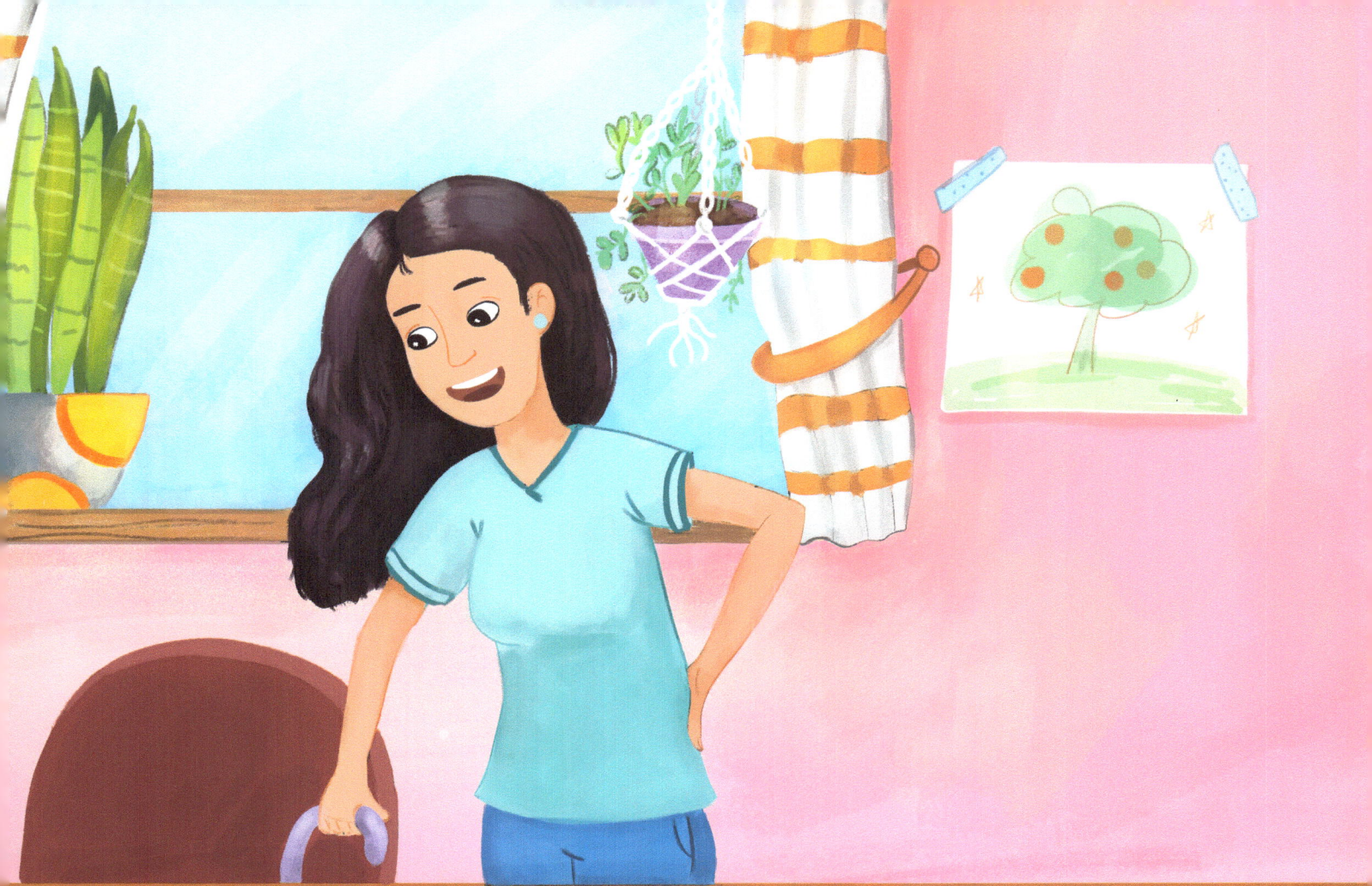

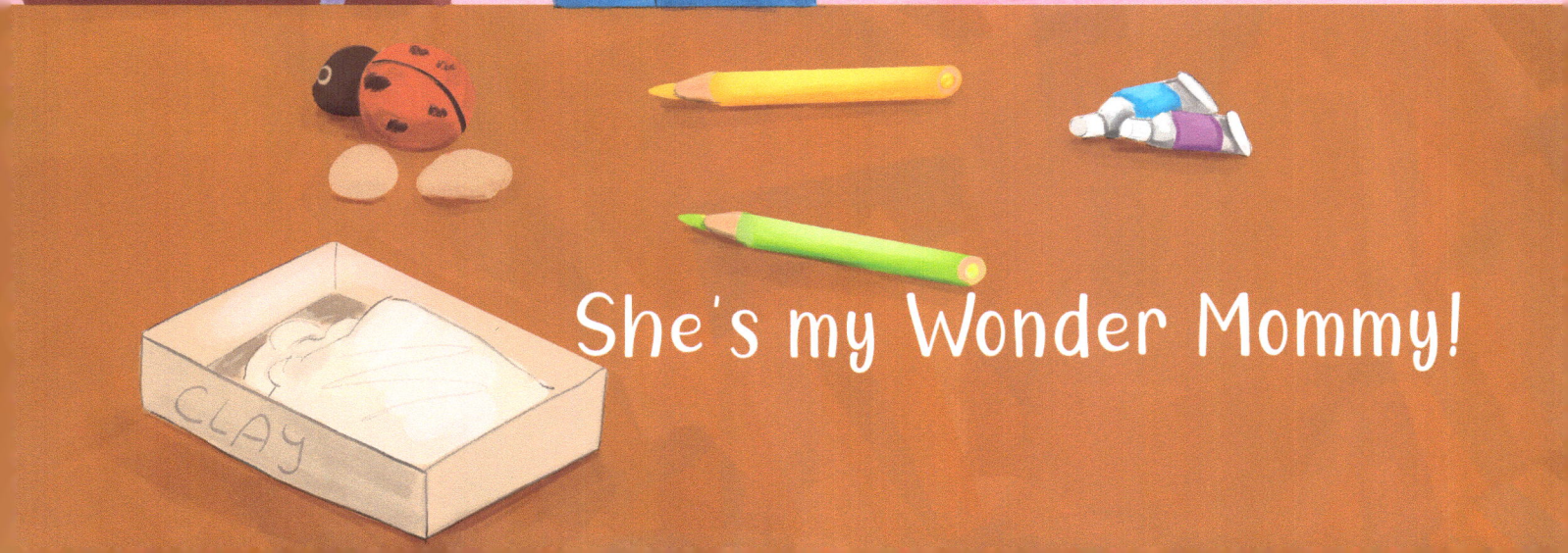

She's my Wonder Mommy!

Mommy loves talking to me.
Sometimes we can be a little noisy.

I share my dreams
and tales from school.
She cheers me on!
My Mommy's cool!

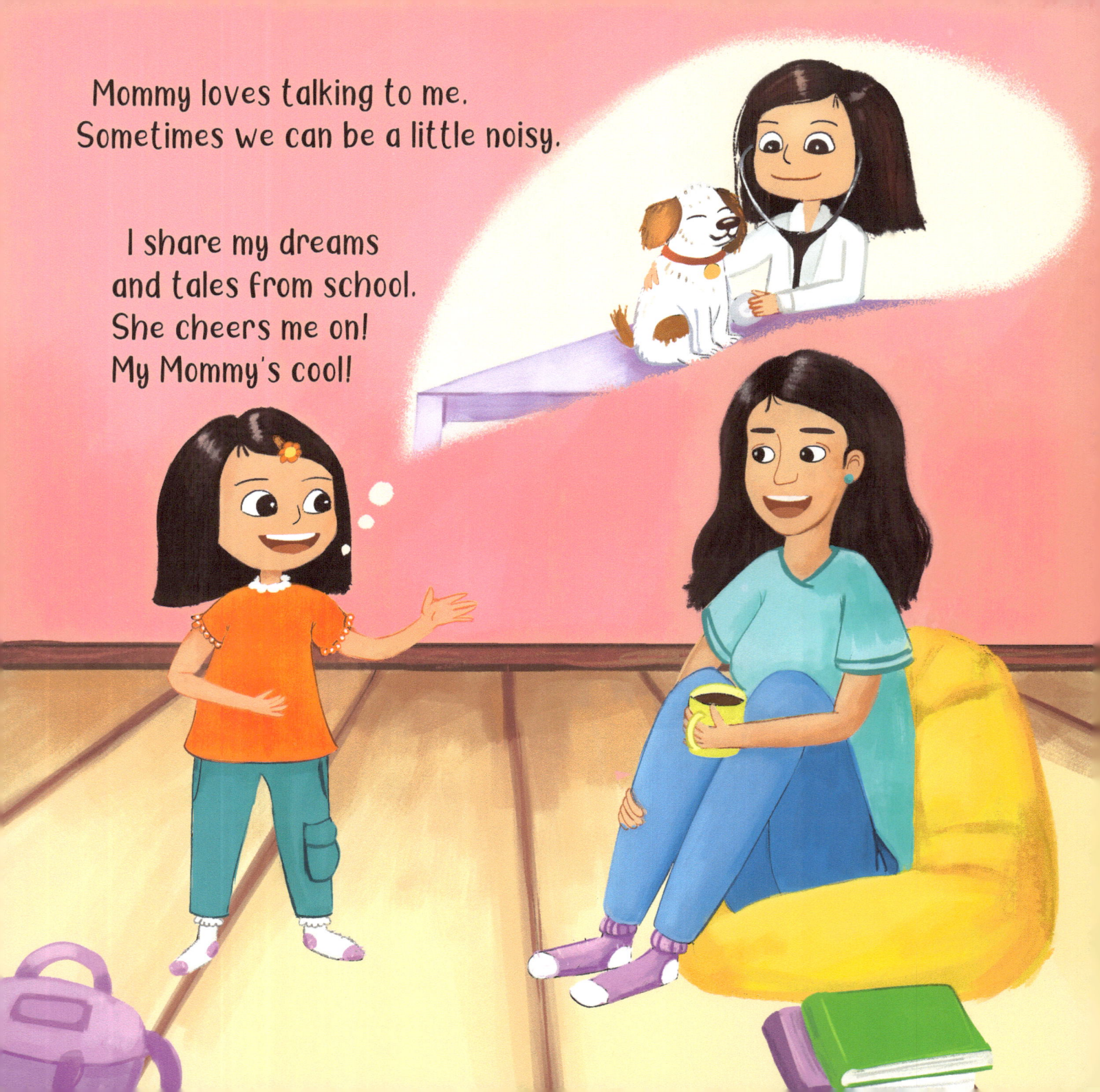

She's my Wonder Mommy!

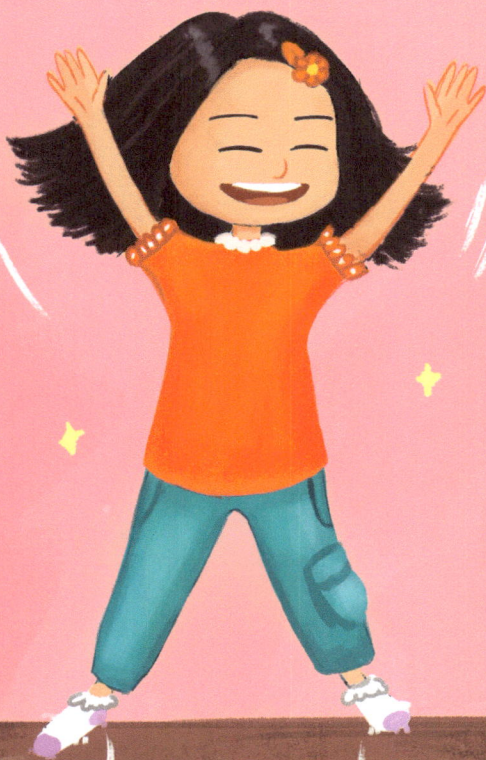

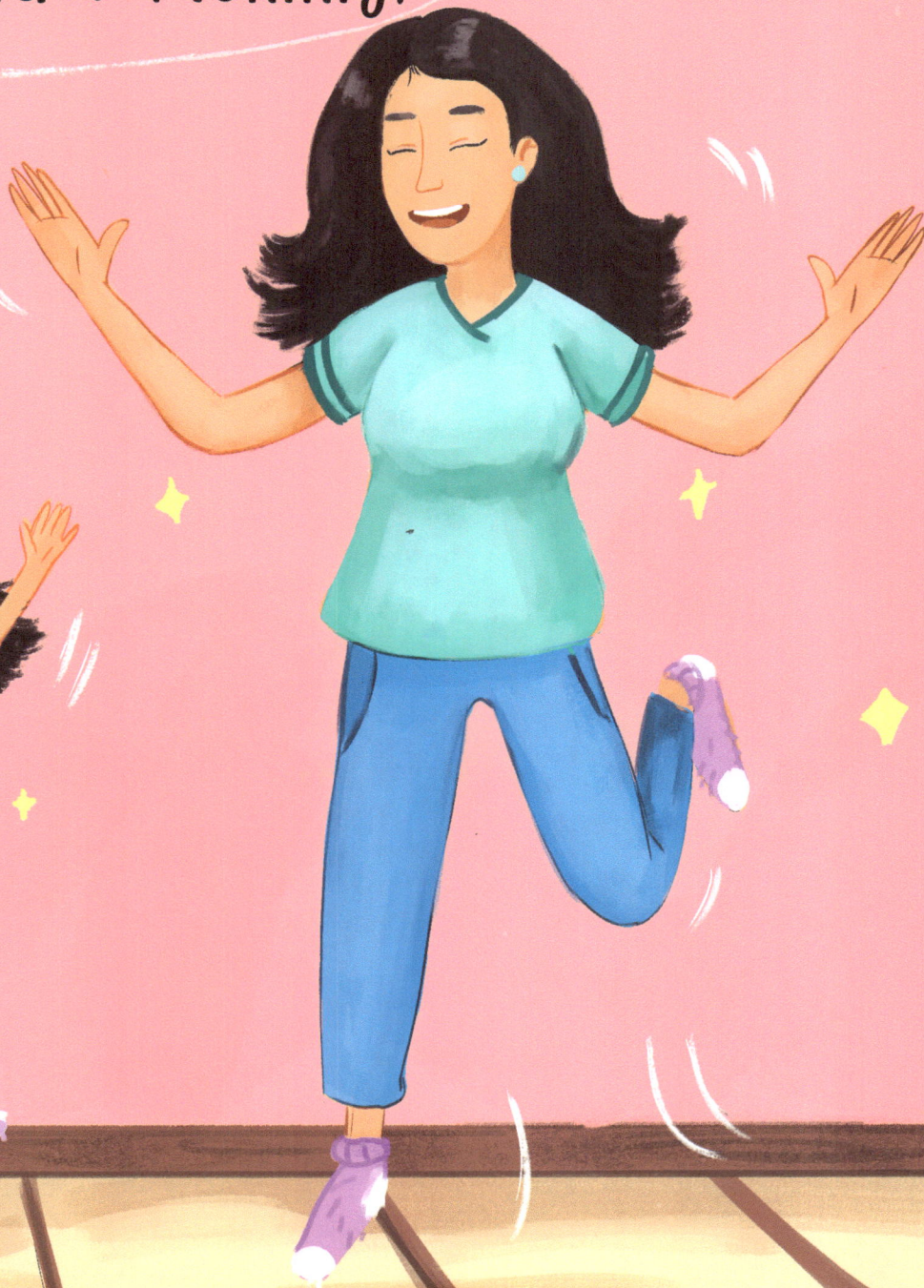

Some days, it's hard for mommy to talk,
so we play quiet games.

We play sink the ship!
We play count the spots!
We play tic tac toe,
and connect the dots!

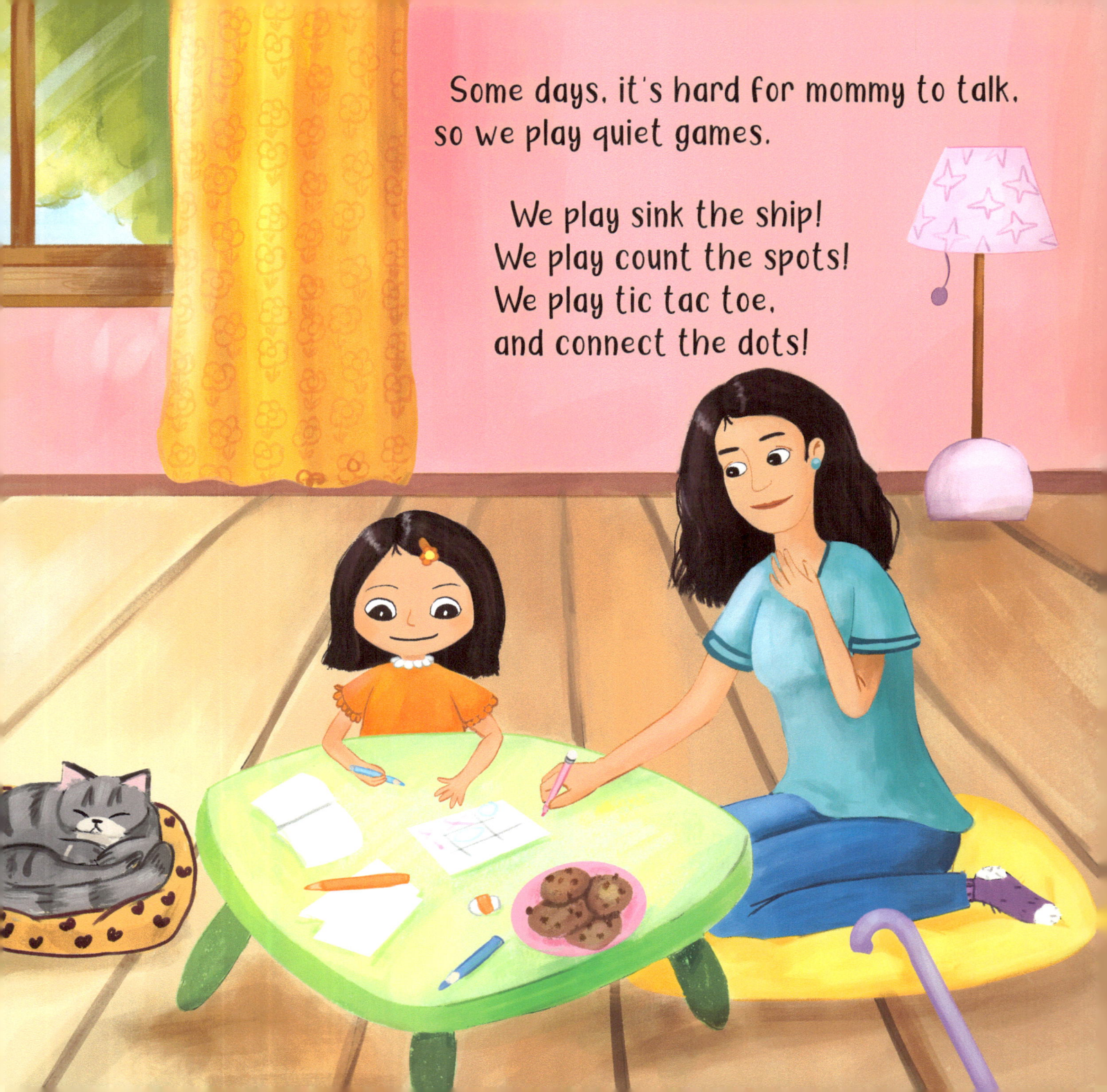

She's my Wonder Mommy!

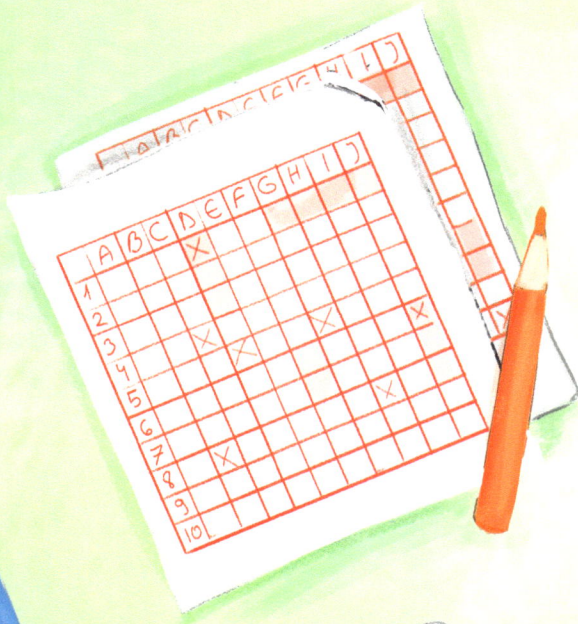

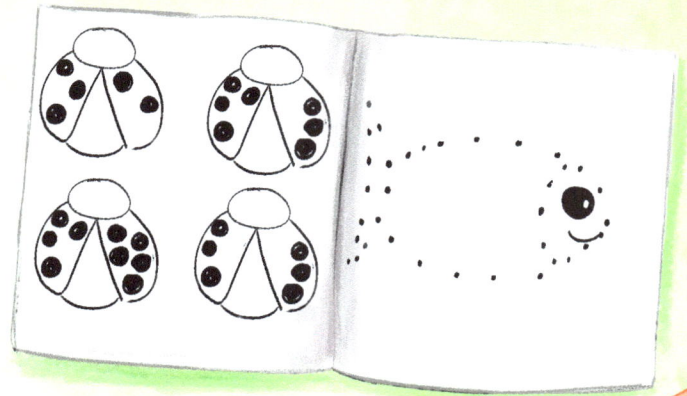

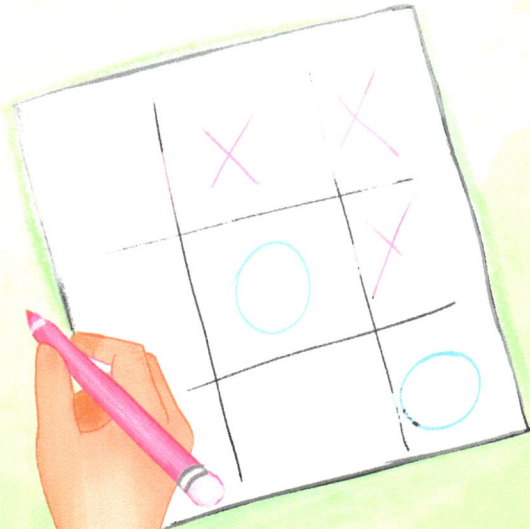

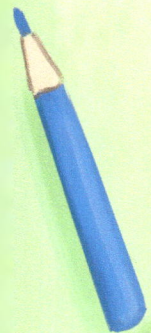

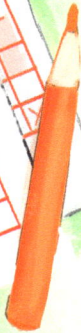

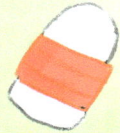

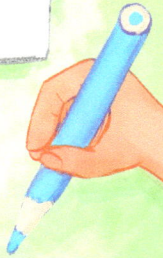

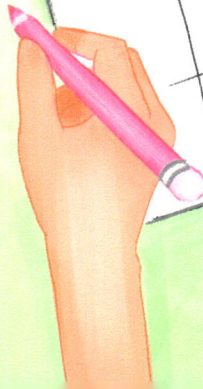

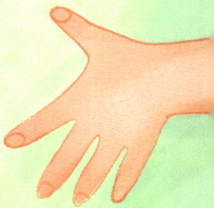

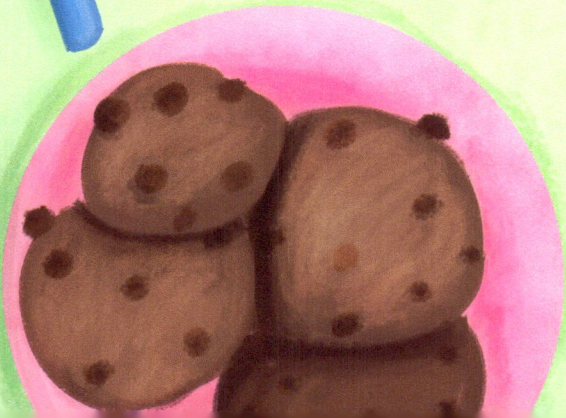

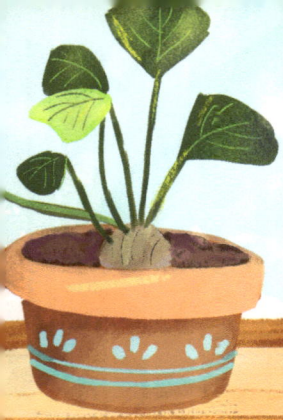

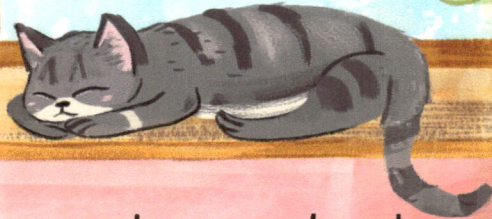

Even though some days are tough,
Mommy finds ways to make me laugh.

She acts like a clown!
We play hide and seek!
Mommy tickles me!
'Mommy, you can't peek!'

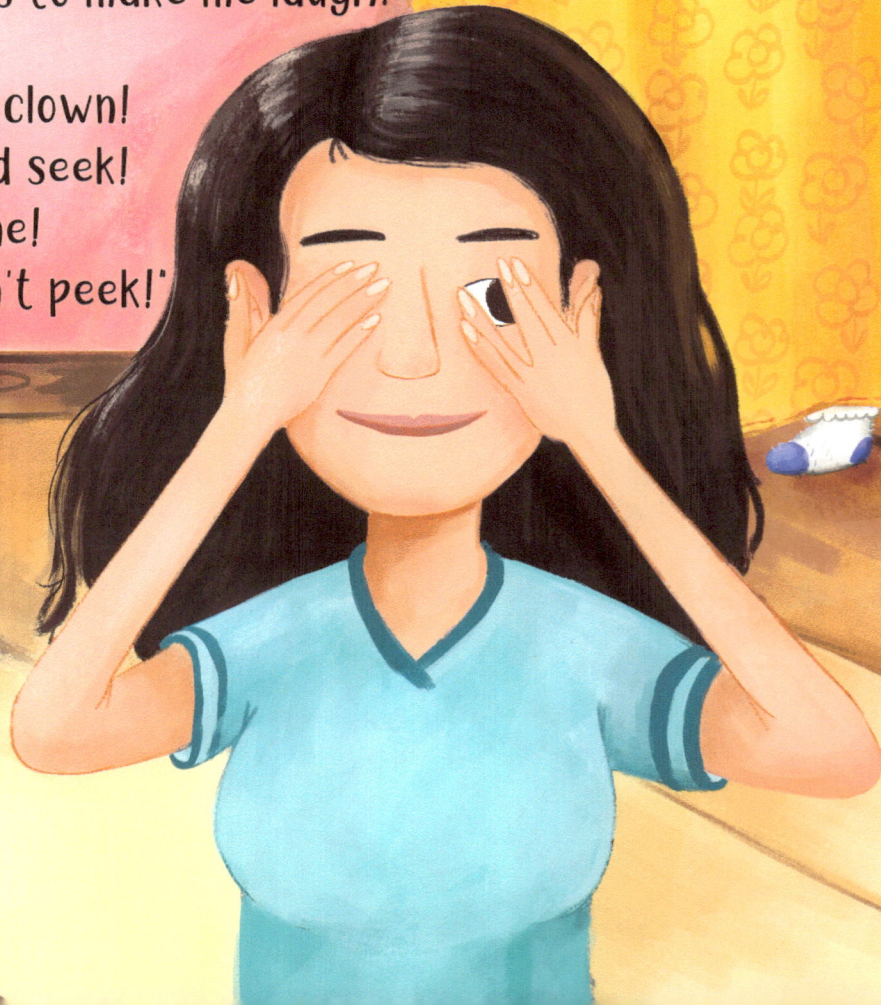

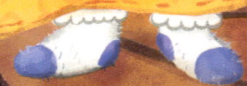

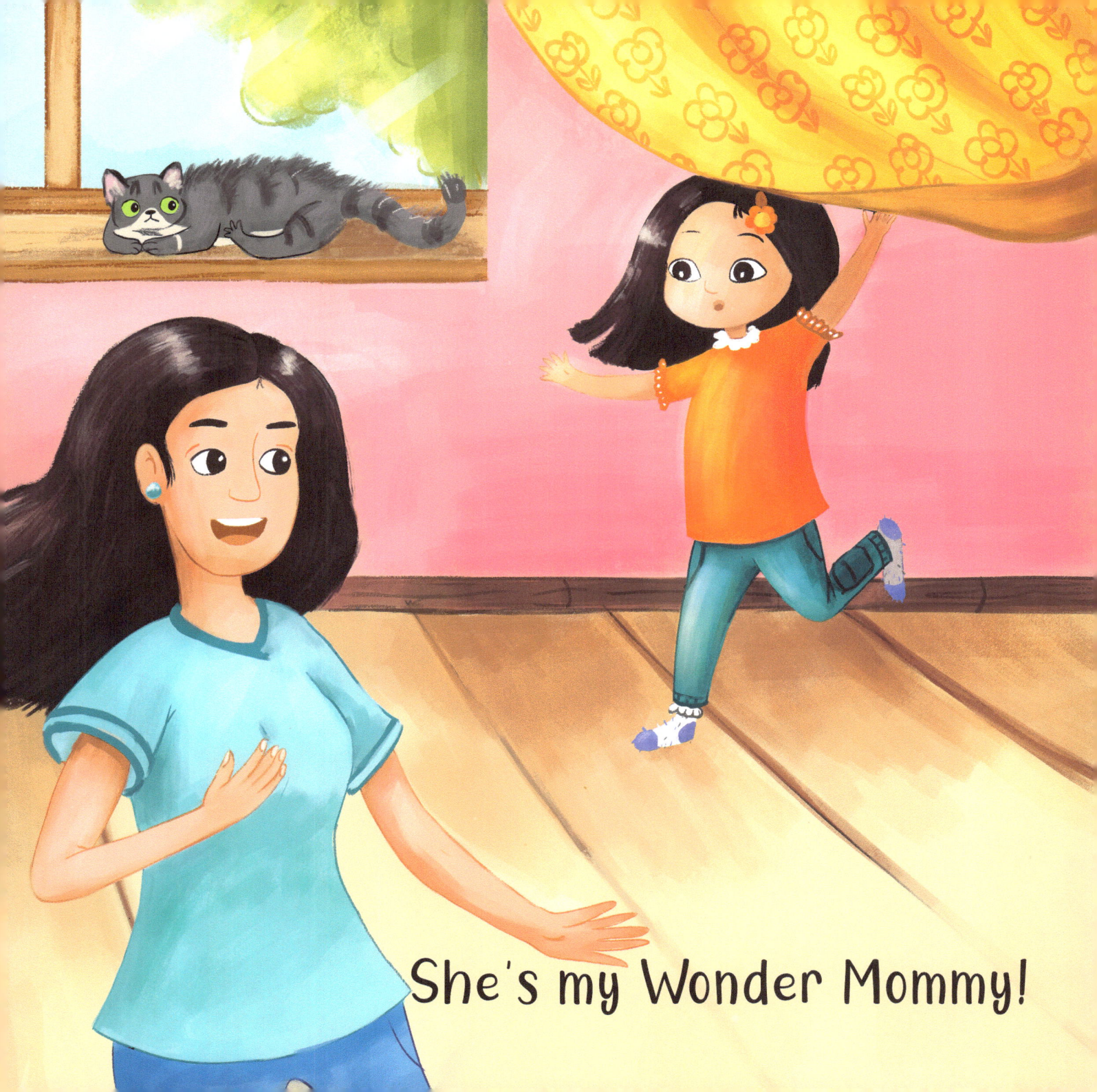

She's my Wonder Mommy!

But there are days when Mommy can't play with me.
Mommy's muscles get stiff and tight, so Daddy
and I stay by her side.

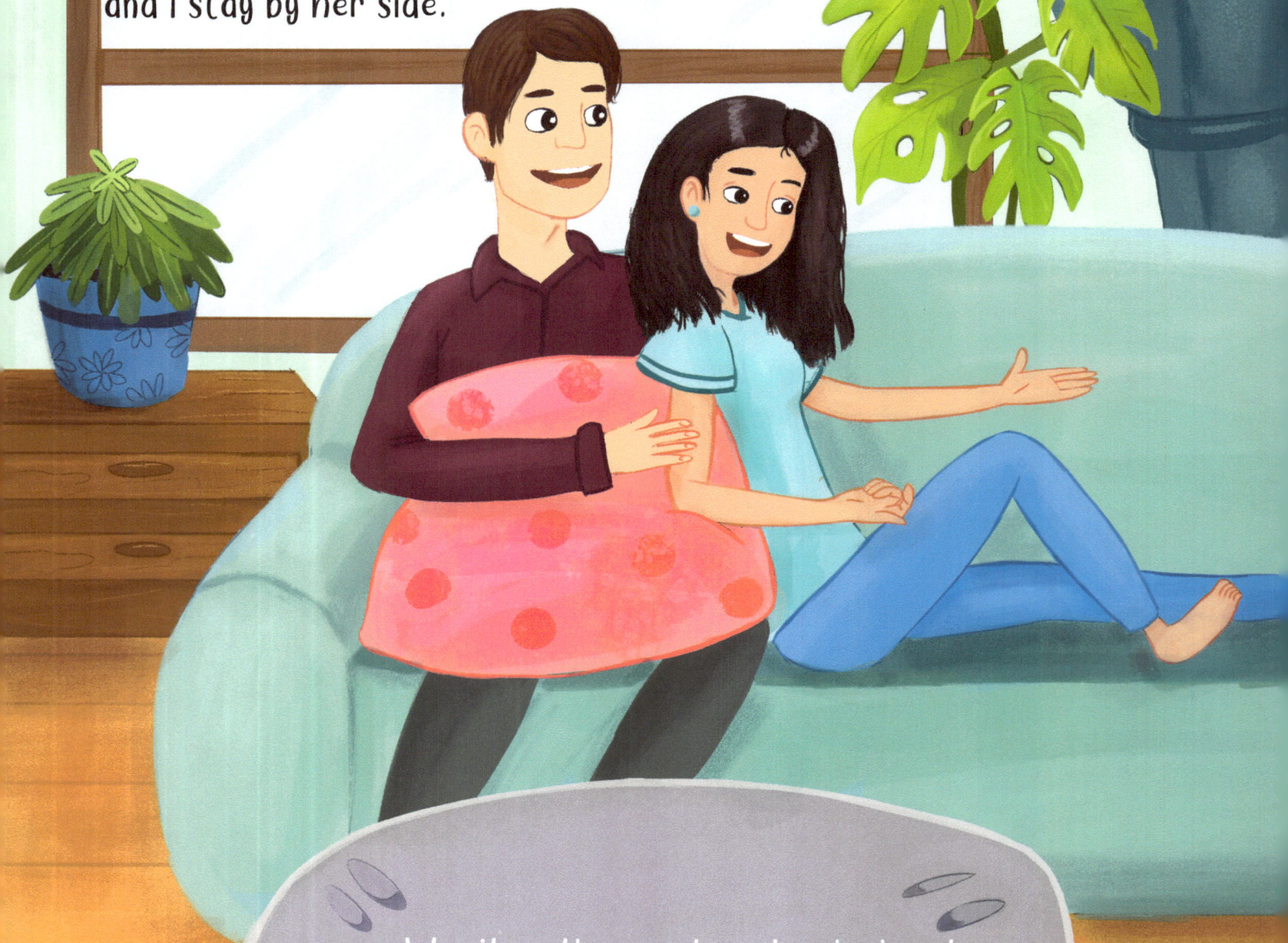

We sit on the couch and make her tea.
We cuddle in bed, and watch TV!

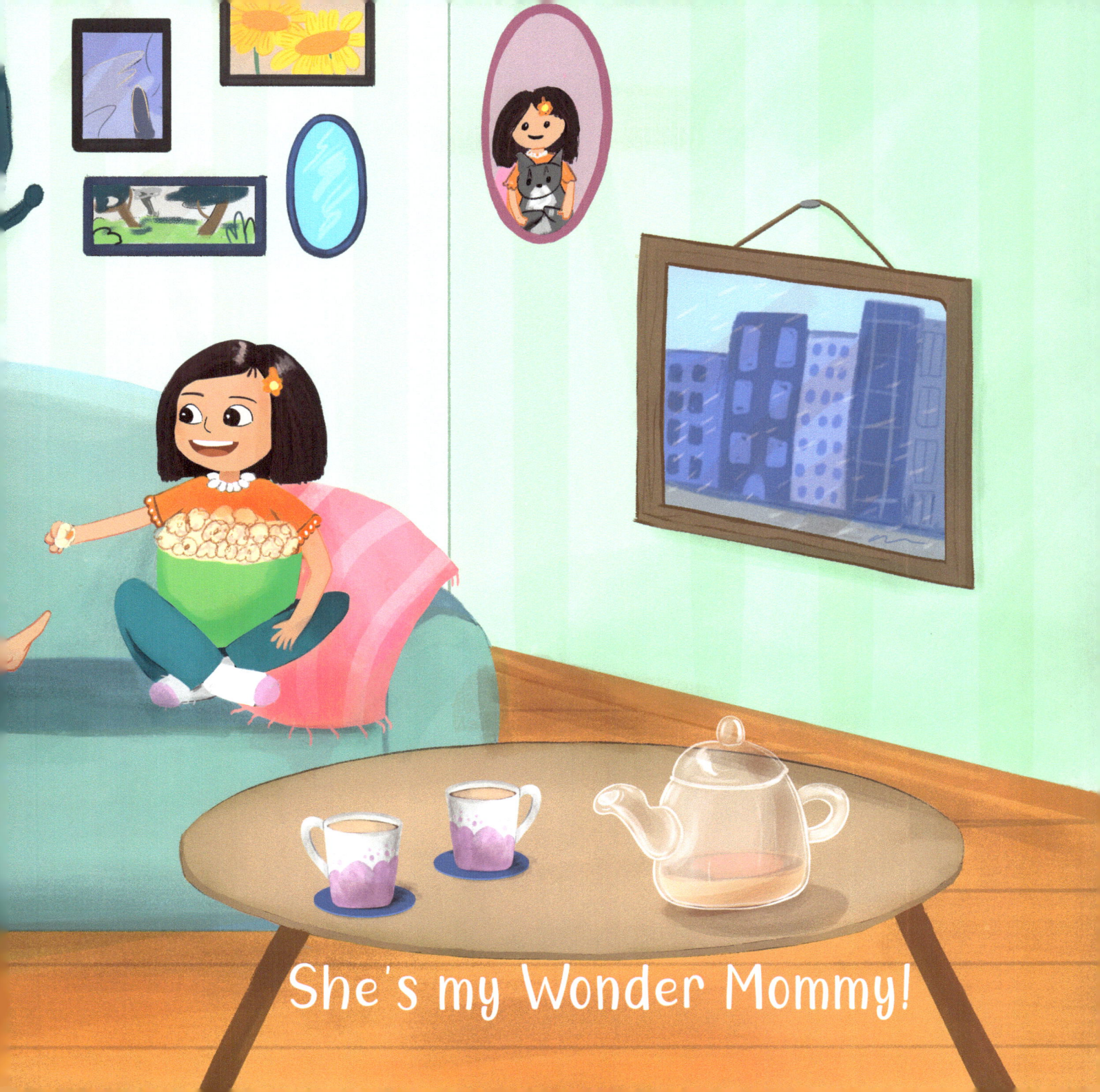

She's my Wonder Mommy!

When Mommy's having a good day, we explore exciting new places!

We go to the beach!
We visit the zoo!
We go to the park!
We go camping too!

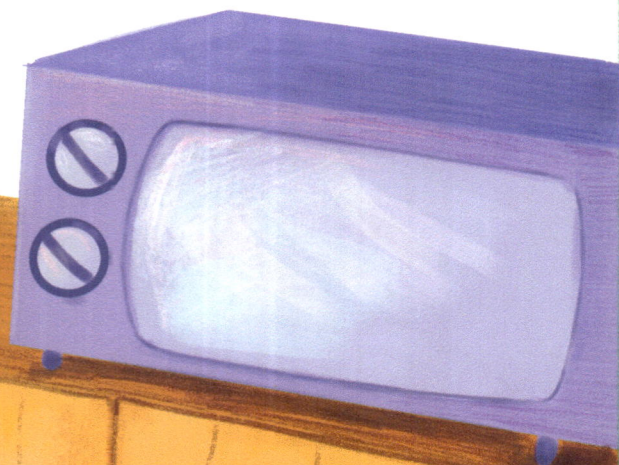

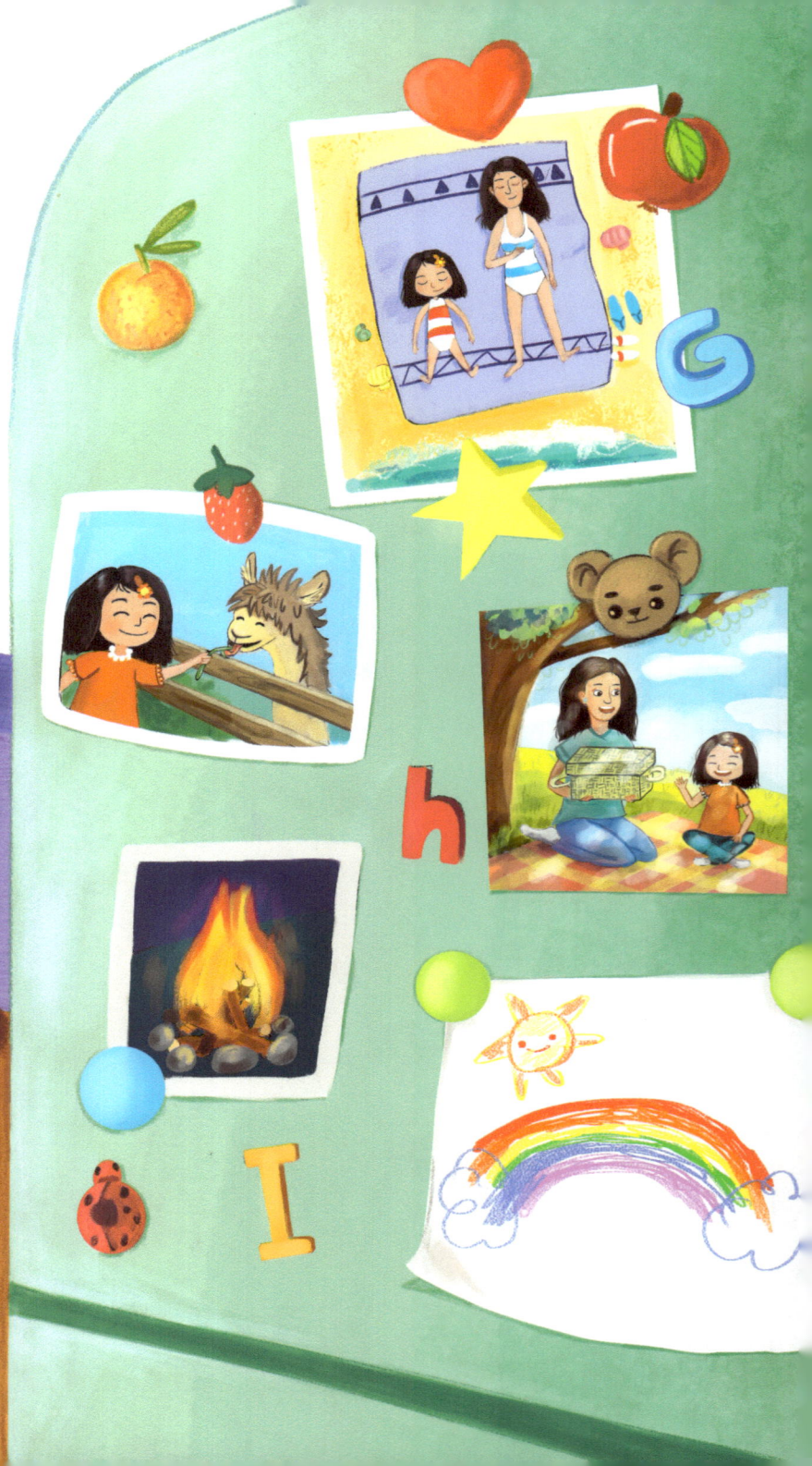

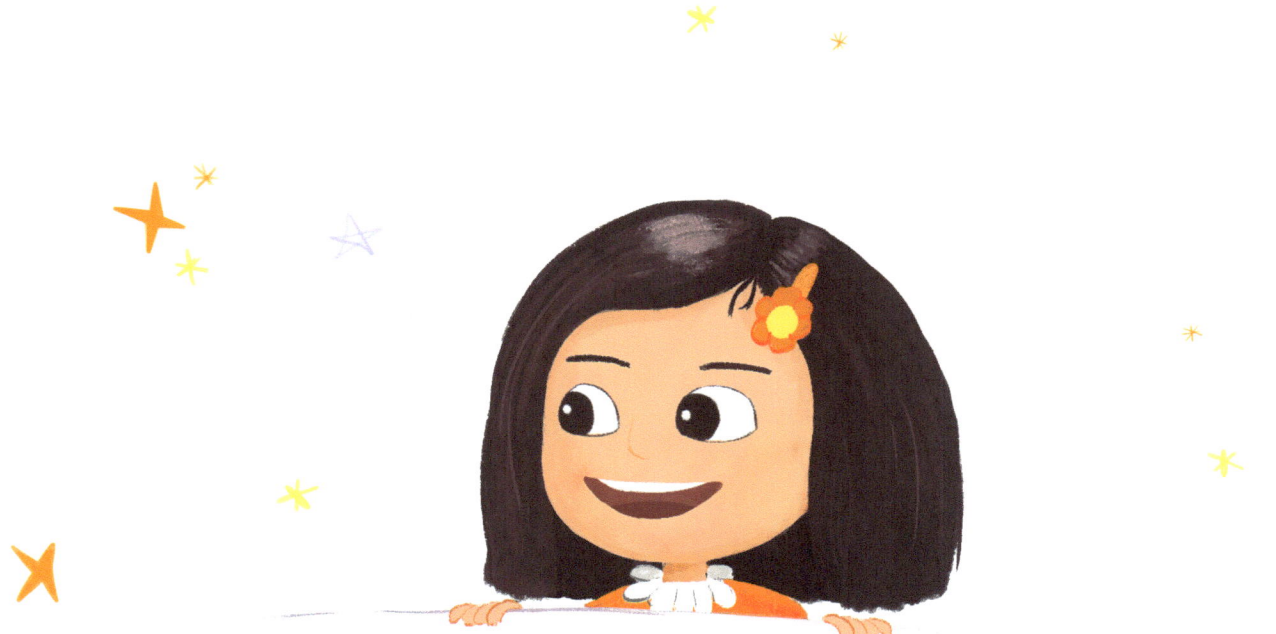

She's my Wonder Mommy!

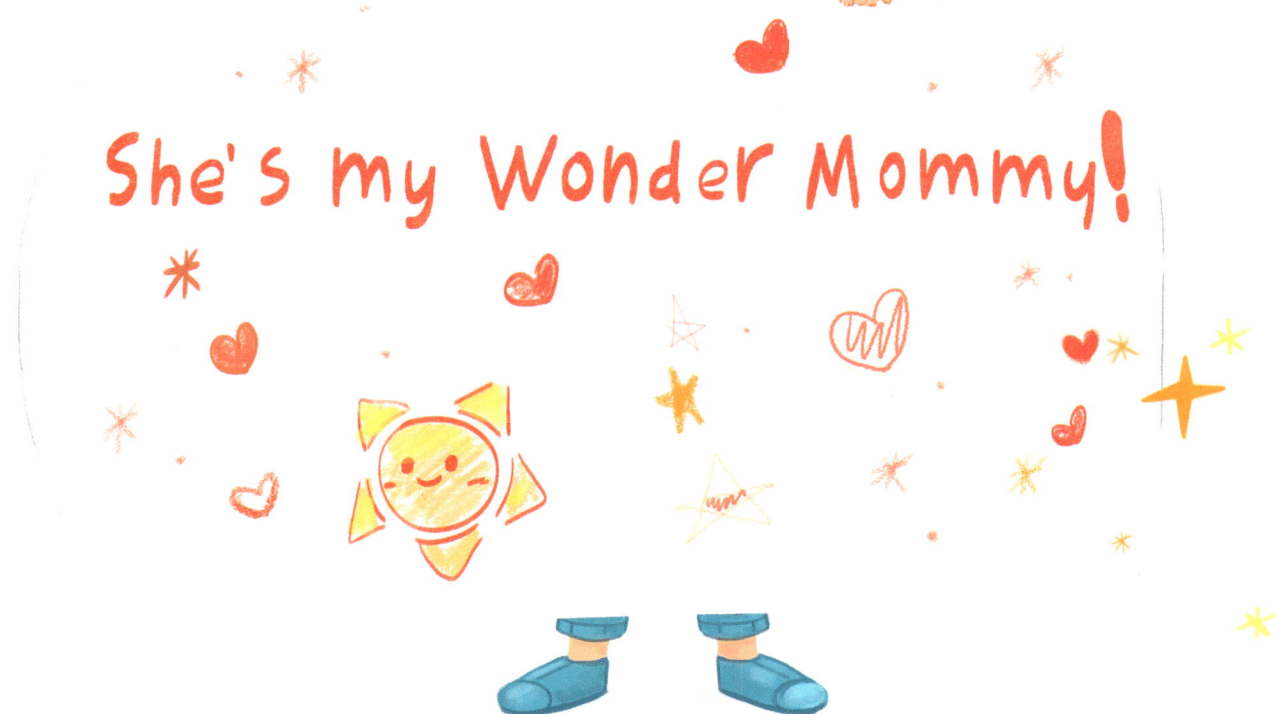

There are days when Mommy really can't go anywhere.

Meow

Her body does things she can't control.
When Mommy is having a rough day,
we stay home and help her feel better.

She takes her medicine,
and I give her a hug.
Kula cuddles with her
'Thank you, my ladybug!'

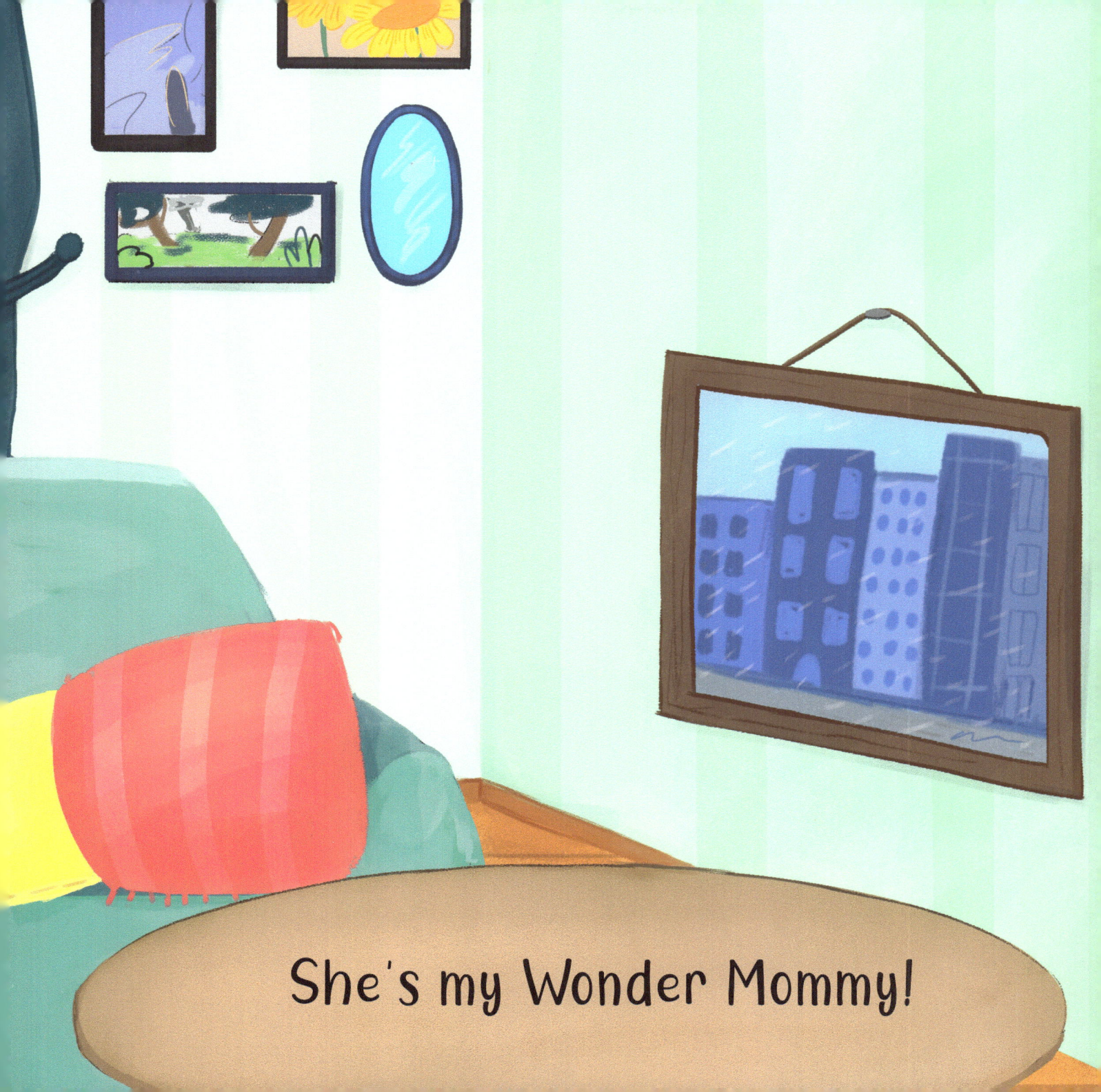

She's my Wonder Mommy!

When Mommy is back on her feet, nothing can stop her.
She goes to the gym!

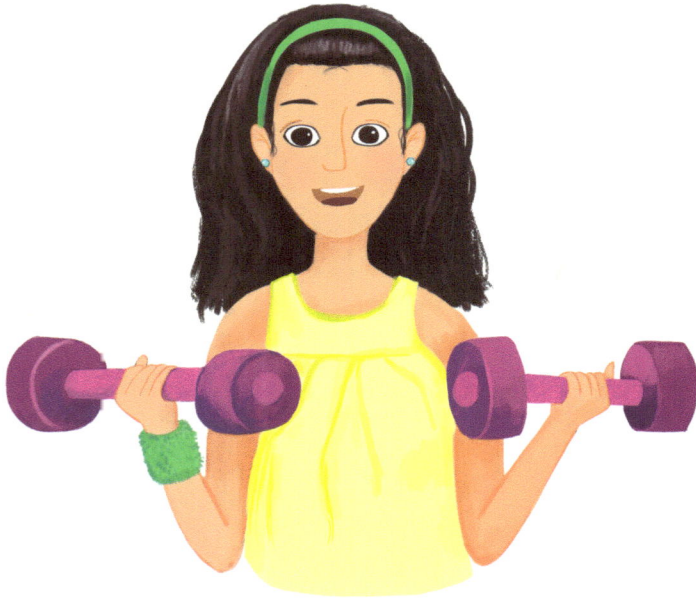

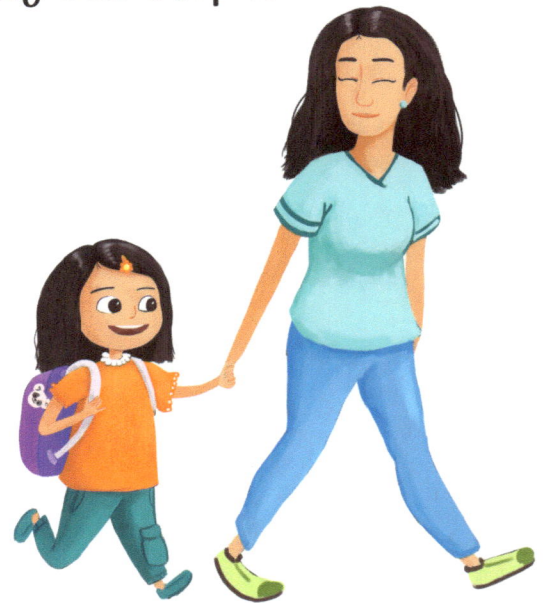

She takes me to school!

She bakes me a cake!

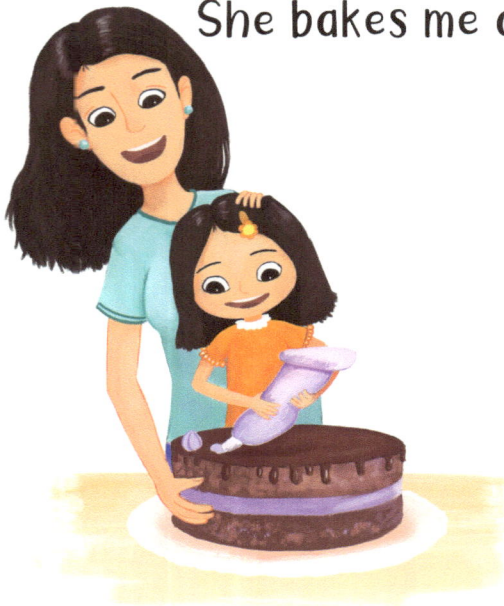

We swim in the pool!

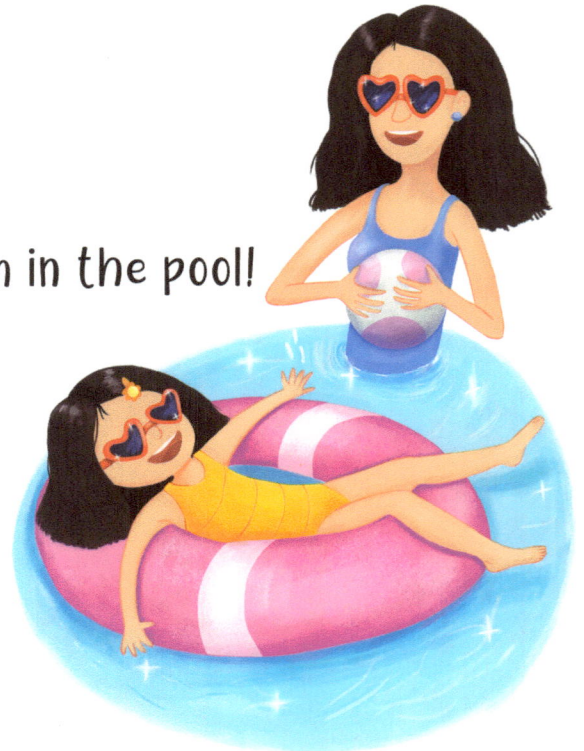

She's my Wonder Mommy!

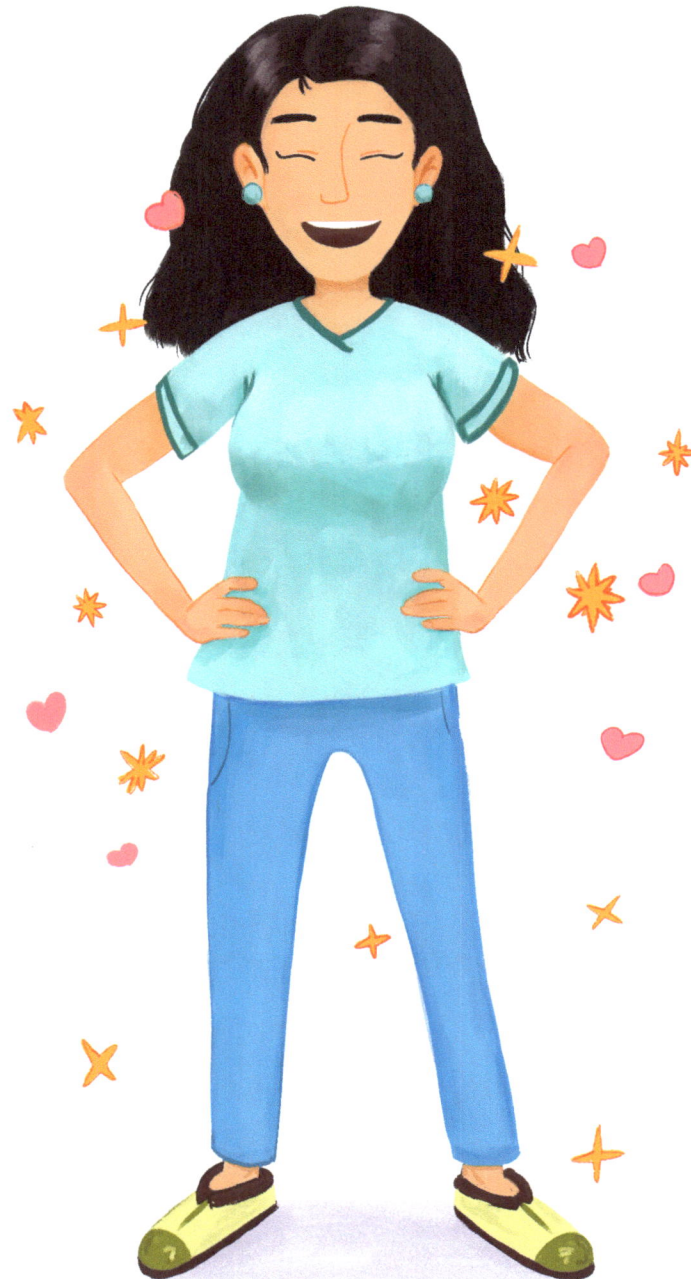

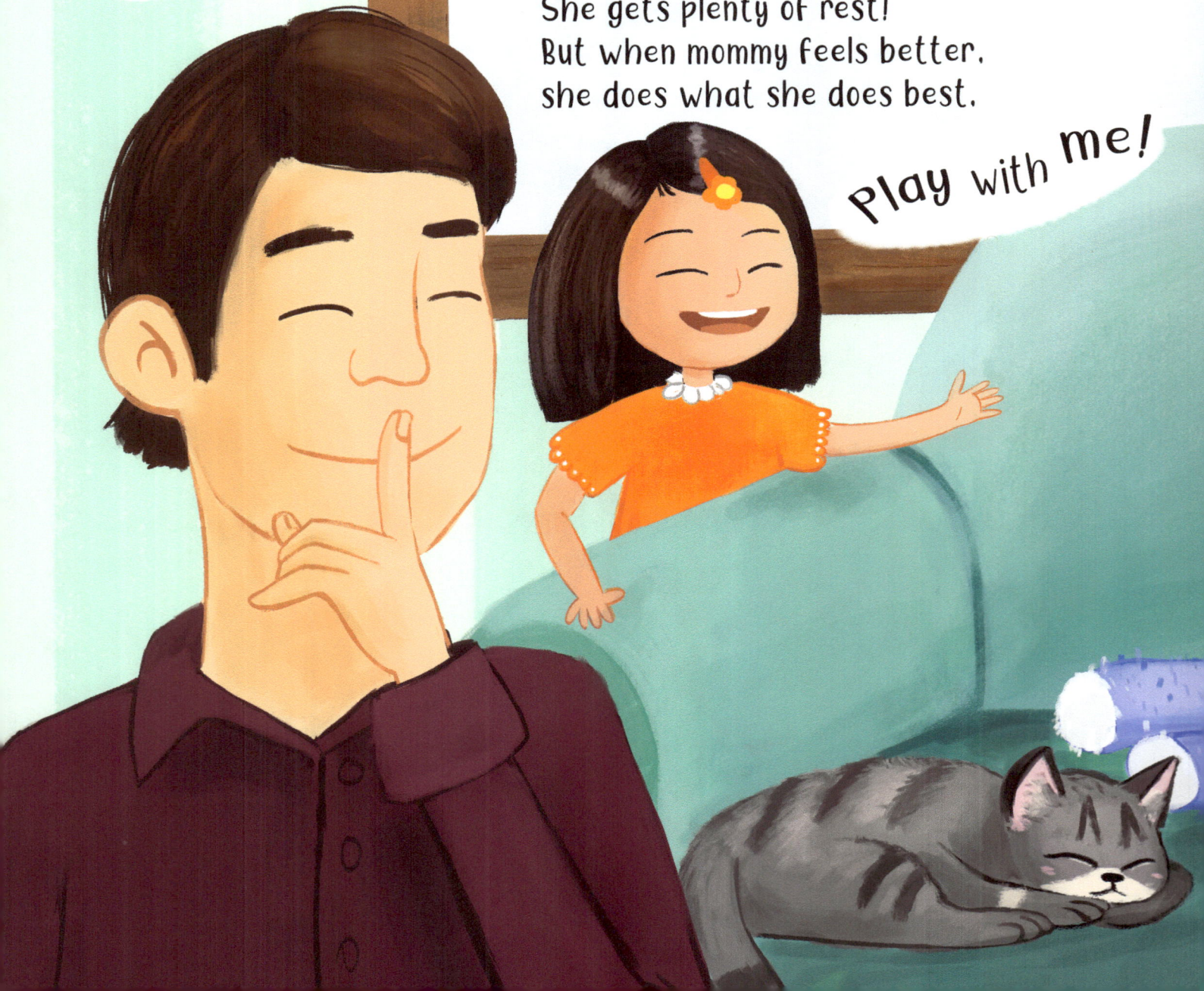

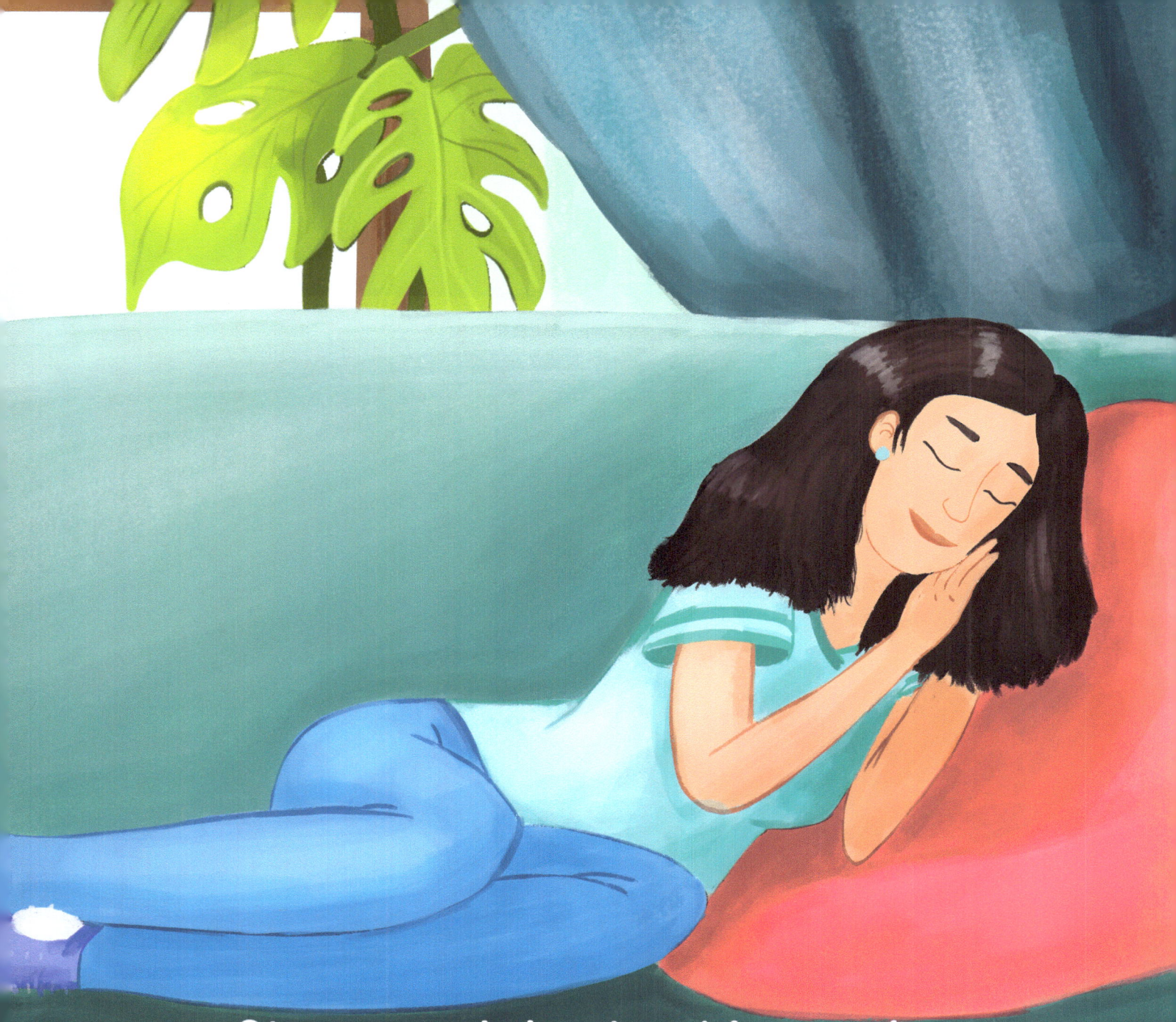

She's my Wonder Mommy!

My mommy is brave.

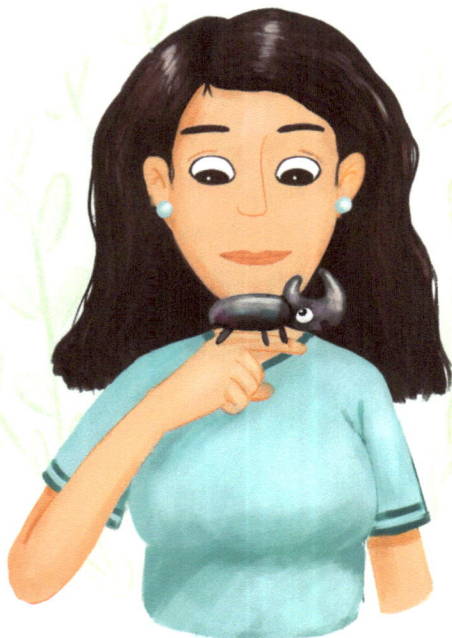

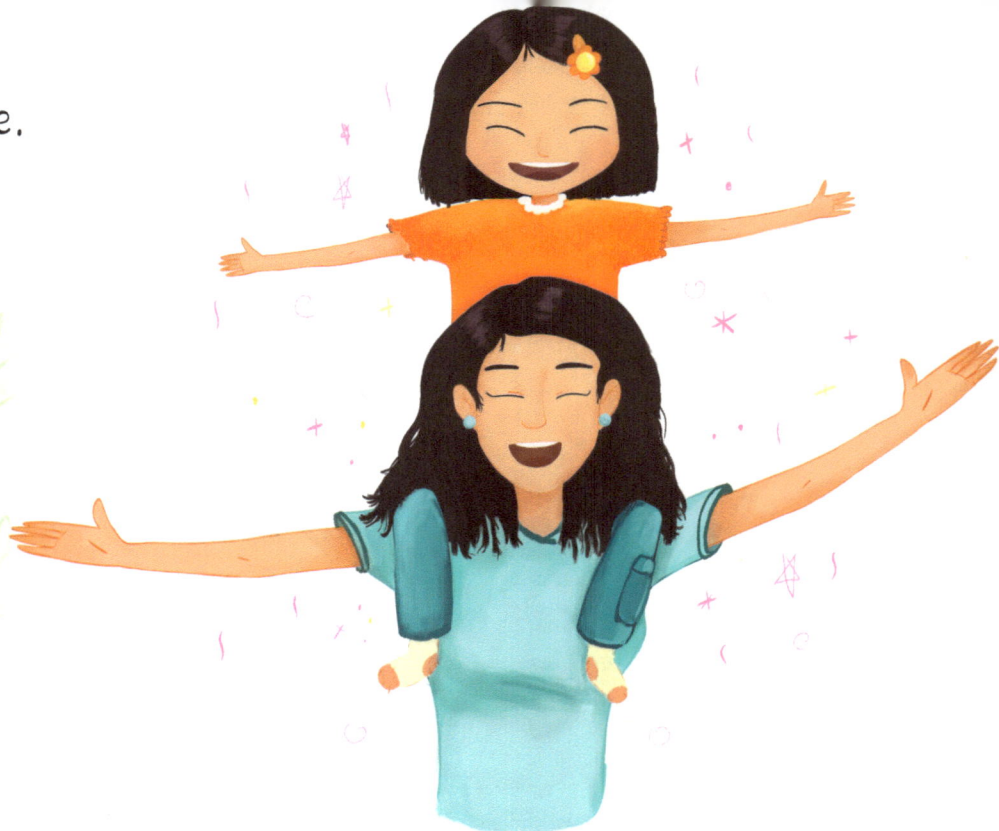

My mommy is strong.

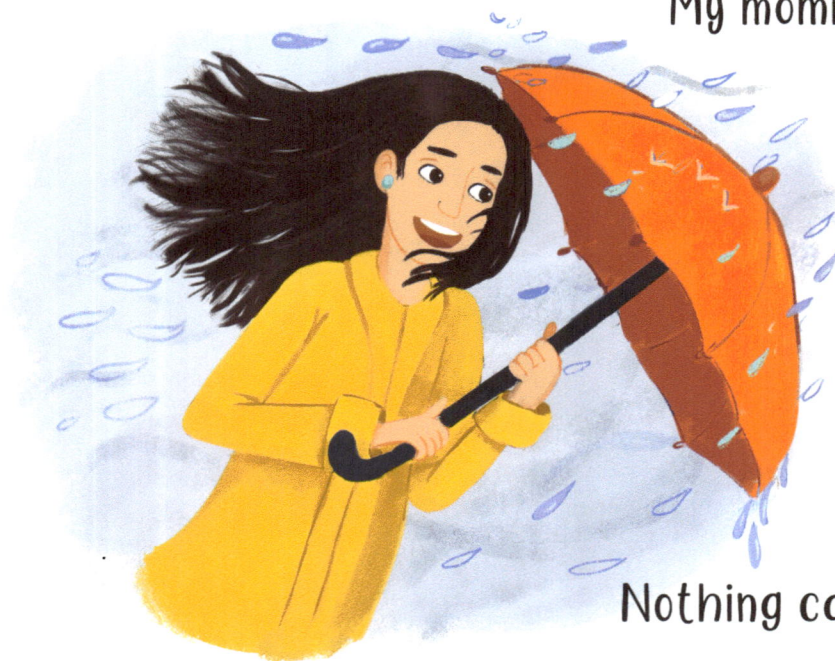

Nothing can defeat her!

I love my Wonder Mommy!

"...and I love you!"

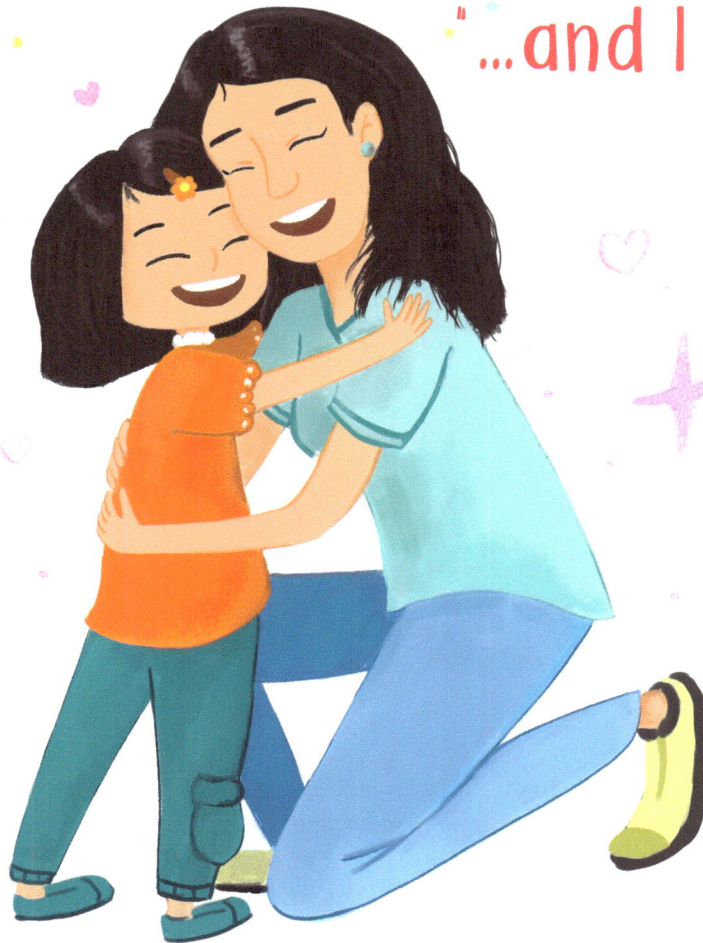

- According to the World Health Organization migraine is one of the ten most disabling medical illnesses on earth.
- Migraine is more than just a headache.

For more information about Migraines, please visit:
https://americanmigrainefoundation.org
https://www.facebook.com/InternationalHemiplegicMigraineFoundation
https://migraine.com/

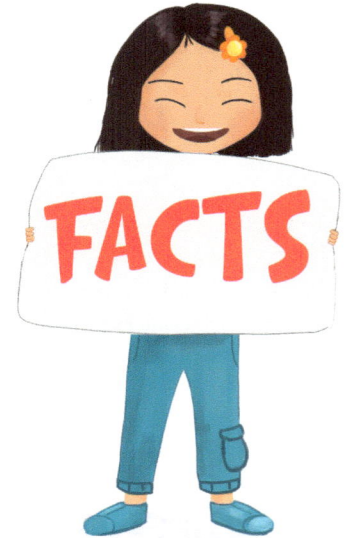

- Dystonia is a neurological disorder that causes excessive, involuntary muscle contractions.
- Dystonia can affect any region of the body including the eyelids, face, jaw, neck, vocal cords, torso, limbs, hands, and feet.

For more information about dystonia, please visit:
https://dystonia-foundation.org/

About the Author

Jennifer is a wife, a wonder mommy, and a chronic illness warrior!
She resides on the beautiful island of Guam with her husband, her youngest
daughter, Kayla, and her two furry babies, Rondo and Kula. Jennifer is one
of the many people who suffer from the debilitating effects of chronic
illness. After so many years of living with a rare type of migraine called,
hemiplegic migraine and a movement disorder called, dystonia, she found
her voice through writing and speaking openly about the challenges she faces.
Having survived parenting three children while battling chronic illnesses, Jennifer
wants to give other parents hope and encouragement through her book.
Jennifer is passionate about spreading awareness about migraine and dystonia
and hopes to break the stigma associated with the conditions.

Jennifer's other titles, Believe (2017) and Good Morning, Mirror (2019).

www.jennifersenne.com

https://www.facebook.com/authorjennifersenne

https://www.instagram.com/author_jennifersenne

About the Illustror

Andreea Balcan is a freelance illustrator based in Brasov-Transylvania.
Having graduated Master of Fine Arts in Cluj-Napoca and having drawn
too many cats to remember, she discovered a passion for fun and quirky
illustrations that led her to enjoy working on children's books.

THANK YOU